THE PAIN OF PROGRESS IS BETTER THAN THE PAIN OF REGRET."

WEEKLY

Weightloss tracker

STARTING WEIGHT

ENDING WEIGHT

Health Tracker

	WEEKLY MEAL PLAN			WATER INTAKE	WORKOUT/EXERCISE	
SUN	B	cal:	carbs:		STRENGTH	DURATION
	L	cal:	carbs:		CARDIO	MILES
	D	cal:	carbs:			STEP COUNT
	S	cal:	carbs:		FLEXIBILITY	CALORIES BURNT
MON	B	cal:	carbs:		STRENGTH	DURATION
	L	cal:	carbs:		CARDIO	MILES
	D	cal:	carbs:			STEP COUNT
	S	cal:	carbs:		FLEXIBILITY	CALORIES BURNT
TUES	B	cal:	carbs:		STRENGTH	DURATION
	L	cal:	carbs:		CARDIO	MILES
	D	cal:	carbs:			STEP COUNT
	S	cal:	carbs:		FLEXIBILITY	CALORIES BURNT
WED	B	cal:	carbs:		STRENGTH	DURATION
	L	cal:	carbs:		CARDIO	MILES
	D	cal:	carbs:			STEP COUNT
	S	cal:	carbs:		FLEXIBILITY	CALORIES BURNT
THUR	B	cal:	carbs:		STRENGTH	DURATION
	L	cal:	carbs:		CARDIO	MILES
	D	cal:	carbs:			STEP COUNT
	S	cal:	carbs:		FLEXIBILITY	CALORIES BURNT
FRI	B	cal:	carbs:		STRENGTH	DURATION
	L	cal:	carbs:		CARDIO	MILES
	D	cal:	carbs:			STEP COUNT
	S	cal:	carbs:		FLEXIBILITY	CALORIES BURNT
SAT	B	cal:	carbs:		STRENGTH	DURATION
	L	cal:	carbs:		CARDIO	MILES
	D	cal:	carbs:			STEP COUNT
	S	cal:	carbs:		FLEXIBILITY	CALORIES BURNT

Health Tracker

	WEEKLY MEAL PLAN			WATER INTAKE	WORKOUT/EXERCISE	
SUN	B	cal:	carbs:		STRENGTH	DURATION
	L	cal:	carbs:			MILES
	D	cal:	carbs:		CARDIO	STEP COUNT
	S	cal:	carbs:		FLEXIBILITY	CALORIES BURNT
MON	B	cal:	carbs:		STRENGTH	DURATION
	L	cal:	carbs:			MILES
	D	cal:	carbs:		CARDIO	STEP COUNT
	S	cal:	carbs:		FLEXIBILITY	CALORIES BURNT
TUES	B	cal:	carbs:		STRENGTH	DURATION
	L	cal:	carbs:			MILES
	D	cal:	carbs:		CARDIO	STEP COUNT
	S	cal:	carbs:		FLEXIBILITY	CALORIES BURNT
WED	B	cal:	carbs:		STRENGTH	DURATION
	L	cal:	carbs:			MILES
	D	cal:	carbs:		CARDIO	STEP COUNT
	S	cal:	carbs:		FLEXIBILITY	CALORIES BURNT
THUR	B	cal:	carbs:		STRENGTH	DURATION
	L	cal:	carbs:			MILES
	D	cal:	carbs:		CARDIO	STEP COUNT
	S	cal:	carbs:		FLEXIBILITY	CALORIES BURNT
FRI	B	cal:	carbs:		STRENGTH	DURATION
	L	cal:	carbs:			MILES
	D	cal:	carbs:		CARDIO	STEP COUNT
	S	cal:	carbs:		FLEXIBILITY	CALORIES BURNT
SAT	B	cal:	carbs:		STRENGTH	DURATION
	L	cal:	carbs:			MILES
	D	cal:	carbs:		CARDIO	STEP COUNT
	S	cal:	carbs:		FLEXIBILITY	CALORIES BURNT

Health Tracker

	WEEKLY MEAL PLAN			WATER INTAKE	WORKOUT/EXERCISE	
SUN	B	cal:	carbs:		STRENGTH	DURATION
	L	cal:	carbs:		CARDIO	MILES
	D	cal:	carbs:			STEP COUNT
	S	cal:	carbs:		FLEXIBILITY	CALORIES BURNT
MON	B	cal:	carbs:		STRENGTH	DURATION
	L	cal:	carbs:		CARDIO	MILES
	D	cal:	carbs:			STEP COUNT
	S	cal:	carbs:		FLEXIBILITY	CALORIES BURNT
TUES	B	cal:	carbs:		STRENGTH	DURATION
	L	cal:	carbs:		CARDIO	MILES
	D	cal:	carbs:			STEP COUNT
	S	cal:	carbs:		FLEXIBILITY	CALORIES BURNT
WED	B	cal:	carbs:		STRENGTH	DURATION
	L	cal:	carbs:		CARDIO	MILES
	D	cal:	carbs:			STEP COUNT
	S	cal:	carbs:		FLEXIBILITY	CALORIES BURNT
THUR	B	cal:	carbs:		STRENGTH	DURATION
	L	cal:	carbs:		CARDIO	MILES
	D	cal:	carbs:			STEP COUNT
	S	cal:	carbs:		FLEXIBILITY	CALORIES BURNT
FRI	B	cal:	carbs:		STRENGTH	DURATION
	L	cal:	carbs:		CARDIO	MILES
	D	cal:	carbs:			STEP COUNT
	S	cal:	carbs:		FLEXIBILITY	CALORIES BURNT
SAT	B	cal:	carbs:		STRENGTH	DURATION
	L	cal:	carbs:		CARDIO	MILES
	D	cal:	carbs:			STEP COUNT
	S	cal:	carbs:		FLEXIBILITY	CALORIES BURNT

Health Tracker

	WEEKLY MEAL PLAN			WATER INTAKE	WORKOUT/EXERCISE	
SUN	B	cal:	carbs:		STRENGTH	DURATION
	L	cal:	carbs:		CARDIO	MILES
	D	cal:	carbs:			STEP COUNT
	S	cal:	carbs:		FLEXIBILITY	CALORIES BURNT
MON	B	cal:	carbs:		STRENGTH	DURATION
	L	cal:	carbs:		CARDIO	MILES
	D	cal:	carbs:			STEP COUNT
	S	cal:	carbs:		FLEXIBILITY	CALORIES BURNT
TUES	B	cal:	carbs:		STRENGTH	DURATION
	L	cal:	carbs:		CARDIO	MILES
	D	cal:	carbs:			STEP COUNT
	S	cal:	carbs:		FLEXIBILITY	CALORIES BURNT
WED	B	cal:	carbs:		STRENGTH	DURATION
	L	cal:	carbs:		CARDIO	MILES
	D	cal:	carbs:			STEP COUNT
	S	cal:	carbs:		FLEXIBILITY	CALORIES BURNT
THUR	B	cal:	carbs:		STRENGTH	DURATION
	L	cal:	carbs:		CARDIO	MILES
	D	cal:	carbs:			STEP COUNT
	S	cal:	carbs:		FLEXIBILITY	CALORIES BURNT
FRI	B	cal:	carbs:		STRENGTH	DURATION
	L	cal:	carbs:		CARDIO	MILES
	D	cal:	carbs:			STEP COUNT
	S	cal:	carbs:		FLEXIBILITY	CALORIES BURNT
SAT	B	cal:	carbs:		STRENGTH	DURATION
	L	cal:	carbs:		CARDIO	MILES
	D	cal:	carbs:			STEP COUNT
	S	cal:	carbs:		FLEXIBILITY	CALORIES BURNT

"ONE BAD DAY DOESN'T ERASE THE WORK. SHOW UP ANYWAY."

Health Tracker

	WEEKLY MEAL PLAN			WATER INTAKE	WORKOUT/EXERCISE	
SUN	B	cal:	carbs:		STRENGTH	DURATION
	L	cal:	carbs:		CARDIO	MILES
	D	cal:	carbs:			STEP COUNT
	S	cal:	carbs:		FLEXIBILITY	CALORIES BURNT
MON	B	cal:	carbs:		STRENGTH	DURATION
	L	cal:	carbs:		CARDIO	MILES
	D	cal:	carbs:			STEP COUNT
	S	cal:	carbs:		FLEXIBILITY	CALORIES BURNT
TUES	B	cal:	carbs:		STRENGTH	DURATION
	L	cal:	carbs:		CARDIO	MILES
	D	cal:	carbs:			STEP COUNT
	S	cal:	carbs:		FLEXIBILITY	CALORIES BURNT
WED	B	cal:	carbs:		STRENGTH	DURATION
	L	cal:	carbs:		CARDIO	MILES
	D	cal:	carbs:			STEP COUNT
	S	cal:	carbs:		FLEXIBILITY	CALORIES BURNT
THUR	B	cal:	carbs:		STRENGTH	DURATION
	L	cal:	carbs:		CARDIO	MILES
	D	cal:	carbs:			STEP COUNT
	S	cal:	carbs:		FLEXIBILITY	CALORIES BURNT
FRI	B	cal:	carbs:		STRENGTH	DURATION
	L	cal:	carbs:		CARDIO	MILES
	D	cal:	carbs:			STEP COUNT
	S	cal:	carbs:		FLEXIBILITY	CALORIES BURNT
SAT	B	cal:	carbs:		STRENGTH	DURATION
	L	cal:	carbs:		CARDIO	MILES
	D	cal:	carbs:			STEP COUNT
	S	cal:	carbs:		FLEXIBILITY	CALORIES BURNT

Health Tracker

	WEEKLY MEAL PLAN			WATER INTAKE	WORKOUT/EXERCISE	
SUN	B	cal:	carbs:		STRENGTH	DURATION
	L	cal:	carbs:		CARDIO	MILES
	D	cal:	carbs:			STEP COUNT
	S	cal:	carbs:		FLEXIBILITY	CALORIES BURNT
MON	B	cal:	carbs:		STRENGTH	DURATION
	L	cal:	carbs:		CARDIO	MILES
	D	cal:	carbs:			STEP COUNT
	S	cal:	carbs:		FLEXIBILITY	CALORIES BURNT
TUES	B	cal:	carbs:		STRENGTH	DURATION
	L	cal:	carbs:		CARDIO	MILES
	D	cal:	carbs:			STEP COUNT
	S	cal:	carbs:		FLEXIBILITY	CALORIES BURNT
WED	B	cal:	carbs:		STRENGTH	DURATION
	L	cal:	carbs:		CARDIO	MILES
	D	cal:	carbs:			STEP COUNT
	S	cal:	carbs:		FLEXIBILITY	CALORIES BURNT
THUR	B	cal:	carbs:		STRENGTH	DURATION
	L	cal:	carbs:		CARDIO	MILES
	D	cal:	carbs:			STEP COUNT
	S	cal:	carbs:		FLEXIBILITY	CALORIES BURNT
FRI	B	cal:	carbs:		STRENGTH	DURATION
	L	cal:	carbs:		CARDIO	MILES
	D	cal:	carbs:			STEP COUNT
	S	cal:	carbs:		FLEXIBILITY	CALORIES BURNT
SAT	B	cal:	carbs:		STRENGTH	DURATION
	L	cal:	carbs:		CARDIO	MILES
	D	cal:	carbs:			STEP COUNT
	S	cal:	carbs:		FLEXIBILITY	CALORIES BURNT

Health Tracker

Day	WEEKLY MEAL PLAN			WATER INTAKE	WORKOUT/EXERCISE	
SUN	B	cal:	carbs:		STRENGTH	DURATION
	L	cal:	carbs:			MILES
	D	cal:	carbs:		CARDIO	STEP COUNT
	S	cal:	carbs:		FLEXIBILITY	CALORIES BURNT
MON	B	cal:	carbs:		STRENGTH	DURATION
	L	cal:	carbs:			MILES
	D	cal:	carbs:		CARDIO	STEP COUNT
	S	cal:	carbs:		FLEXIBILITY	CALORIES BURNT
TUES	B	cal:	carbs:		STRENGTH	DURATION
	L	cal:	carbs:			MILES
	D	cal:	carbs:		CARDIO	STEP COUNT
	S	cal:	carbs:		FLEXIBILITY	CALORIES BURNT
WED	B	cal:	carbs:		STRENGTH	DURATION
	L	cal:	carbs:			MILES
	D	cal:	carbs:		CARDIO	STEP COUNT
	S	cal:	carbs:		FLEXIBILITY	CALORIES BURNT
THUR	B	cal:	carbs:		STRENGTH	DURATION
	L	cal:	carbs:			MILES
	D	cal:	carbs:		CARDIO	STEP COUNT
	S	cal:	carbs:		FLEXIBILITY	CALORIES BURNT
FRI	B	cal:	carbs:		STRENGTH	DURATION
	L	cal:	carbs:			MILES
	D	cal:	carbs:		CARDIO	STEP COUNT
	S	cal:	carbs:		FLEXIBILITY	CALORIES BURNT
SAT	B	cal:	carbs:		STRENGTH	DURATION
	L	cal:	carbs:			MILES
	D	cal:	carbs:		CARDIO	STEP COUNT
	S	cal:	carbs:		FLEXIBILITY	CALORIES BURNT

Health Tracker

	WEEKLY MEAL PLAN			WATER INTAKE	WORKOUT/EXERCISE	
SUN	B	cal:	carbs:		STRENGTH	DURATION
	L	cal:	carbs:			MILES
	D	cal:	carbs:		CARDIO	STEP COUNT
	S	cal:	carbs:		FLEXIBILITY	CALORIES BURNT
MON	B	cal:	carbs:		STRENGTH	DURATION
	L	cal:	carbs:			MILES
	D	cal:	carbs:		CARDIO	STEP COUNT
	S	cal:	carbs:		FLEXIBILITY	CALORIES BURNT
TUES	B	cal:	carbs:		STRENGTH	DURATION
	L	cal:	carbs:			MILES
	D	cal:	carbs:		CARDIO	STEP COUNT
	S	cal:	carbs:		FLEXIBILITY	CALORIES BURNT
WED	B	cal:	carbs:		STRENGTH	DURATION
	L	cal:	carbs:			MILES
	D	cal:	carbs:		CARDIO	STEP COUNT
	S	cal:	carbs:		FLEXIBILITY	CALORIES BURNT
THUR	B	cal:	carbs:		STRENGTH	DURATION
	L	cal:	carbs:			MILES
	D	cal:	carbs:		CARDIO	STEP COUNT
	S	cal:	carbs:		FLEXIBILITY	CALORIES BURNT
FRI	B	cal:	carbs:		STRENGTH	DURATION
	L	cal:	carbs:			MILES
	D	cal:	carbs:		CARDIO	STEP COUNT
	S	cal:	carbs:		FLEXIBILITY	CALORIES BURNT
SAT	B	cal:	carbs:		STRENGTH	DURATION
	L	cal:	carbs:			MILES
	D	cal:	carbs:		CARDIO	STEP COUNT
	S	cal:	carbs:		FLEXIBILITY	CALORIES BURNT

WHAT DIDN'T GO AS PLANNED, AND HOW WILL I ATTACK IT NEXT WEEK?

Health Tracker

	WEEKLY MEAL PLAN			WATER INTAKE	WORKOUT/EXERCISE	
SUN	B	cal:	carbs:		STRENGTH	DURATION
	L	cal:	carbs:		CARDIO	MILES
	D	cal:	carbs:			STEP COUNT
	S	cal:	carbs:		FLEXIBILITY	CALORIES BURNT
MON	B	cal:	carbs:		STRENGTH	DURATION
	L	cal:	carbs:		CARDIO	MILES
	D	cal:	carbs:			STEP COUNT
	S	cal:	carbs:		FLEXIBILITY	CALORIES BURNT
TUES	B	cal:	carbs:		STRENGTH	DURATION
	L	cal:	carbs:		CARDIO	MILES
	D	cal:	carbs:			STEP COUNT
	S	cal:	carbs:		FLEXIBILITY	CALORIES BURNT
WED	B	cal:	carbs:		STRENGTH	DURATION
	L	cal:	carbs:		CARDIO	MILES
	D	cal:	carbs:			STEP COUNT
	S	cal:	carbs:		FLEXIBILITY	CALORIES BURNT
THUR	B	cal:	carbs:		STRENGTH	DURATION
	L	cal:	carbs:		CARDIO	MILES
	D	cal:	carbs:			STEP COUNT
	S	cal:	carbs:		FLEXIBILITY	CALORIES BURNT
FRI	B	cal:	carbs:		STRENGTH	DURATION
	L	cal:	carbs:		CARDIO	MILES
	D	cal:	carbs:			STEP COUNT
	S	cal:	carbs:		FLEXIBILITY	CALORIES BURNT
SAT	B	cal:	carbs:		STRENGTH	DURATION
	L	cal:	carbs:		CARDIO	MILES
	D	cal:	carbs:			STEP COUNT
	S	cal:	carbs:		FLEXIBILITY	CALORIES BURNT

Health Tracker

	WEEKLY MEAL PLAN			WATER INTAKE	WORKOUT/EXERCISE	
SUN	B	cal:	carbs:		STRENGTH	DURATION
	L	cal:	carbs:		CARDIO	MILES
	D	cal:	carbs:			STEP COUNT
	S	cal:	carbs:		FLEXIBILITY	CALORIES BURNT
MON	B	cal:	carbs:		STRENGTH	DURATION
	L	cal:	carbs:		CARDIO	MILES
	D	cal:	carbs:			STEP COUNT
	S	cal:	carbs:		FLEXIBILITY	CALORIES BURNT
TUES	B	cal:	carbs:		STRENGTH	DURATION
	L	cal:	carbs:		CARDIO	MILES
	D	cal:	carbs:			STEP COUNT
	S	cal:	carbs:		FLEXIBILITY	CALORIES BURNT
WED	B	cal:	carbs:		STRENGTH	DURATION
	L	cal:	carbs:		CARDIO	MILES
	D	cal:	carbs:			STEP COUNT
	S	cal:	carbs:		FLEXIBILITY	CALORIES BURNT
THUR	B	cal:	carbs:		STRENGTH	DURATION
	L	cal:	carbs:		CARDIO	MILES
	D	cal:	carbs:			STEP COUNT
	S	cal:	carbs:		FLEXIBILITY	CALORIES BURNT
FRI	B	cal:	carbs:		STRENGTH	DURATION
	L	cal:	carbs:		CARDIO	MILES
	D	cal:	carbs:			STEP COUNT
	S	cal:	carbs:		FLEXIBILITY	CALORIES BURNT
SAT	B	cal:	carbs:		STRENGTH	DURATION
	L	cal:	carbs:		CARDIO	MILES
	D	cal:	carbs:			STEP COUNT
	S	cal:	carbs:		FLEXIBILITY	CALORIES BURNT

START OVER IF YOU MUST, JUST NEVER GIVE UP.

Health Tracker

	WEEKLY MEAL PLAN			WATER INTAKE	WORKOUT/EXERCISE	
SUN	B	cal:	carbs:		STRENGTH	DURATION
	L	cal:	carbs:			MILES
	D	cal:	carbs:		CARDIO	STEP COUNT
	S	cal:	carbs:		FLEXIBILITY	CALORIES BURNT
MON	B	cal:	carbs:		STRENGTH	DURATION
	L	cal:	carbs:			MILES
	D	cal:	carbs:		CARDIO	STEP COUNT
	S	cal:	carbs:		FLEXIBILITY	CALORIES BURNT
TUES	B	cal:	carbs:		STRENGTH	DURATION
	L	cal:	carbs:			MILES
	D	cal:	carbs:		CARDIO	STEP COUNT
	S	cal:	carbs:		FLEXIBILITY	CALORIES BURNT
WED	B	cal:	carbs:		STRENGTH	DURATION
	L	cal:	carbs:			MILES
	D	cal:	carbs:		CARDIO	STEP COUNT
	S	cal:	carbs:		FLEXIBILITY	CALORIES BURNT
THUR	B	cal:	carbs:		STRENGTH	DURATION
	L	cal:	carbs:			MILES
	D	cal:	carbs:		CARDIO	STEP COUNT
	S	cal:	carbs:		FLEXIBILITY	CALORIES BURNT
FRI	B	cal:	carbs:		STRENGTH	DURATION
	L	cal:	carbs:			MILES
	D	cal:	carbs:		CARDIO	STEP COUNT
	S	cal:	carbs:		FLEXIBILITY	CALORIES BURNT
SAT	B	cal:	carbs:		STRENGTH	DURATION
	L	cal:	carbs:			MILES
	D	cal:	carbs:		CARDIO	STEP COUNT
	S	cal:	carbs:		FLEXIBILITY	CALORIES BURNT

Health Tracker

	WEEKLY MEAL PLAN			WATER INTAKE	WORKOUT/EXERCISE	
SUN	B	cal:	carbs:		☐ STRENGTH	DURATION
	L	cal:	carbs:		☐ CARDIO	MILES
	D	cal:	carbs:			STEP COUNT
	S	cal:	carbs:		☐ FLEXIBILITY	CALORIES BURNT
MON	B	cal:	carbs:		☐ STRENGTH	DURATION
	L	cal:	carbs:		☐ CARDIO	MILES
	D	cal:	carbs:			STEP COUNT
	S	cal:	carbs:		☐ FLEXIBILITY	CALORIES BURNT
TUES	B	cal:	carbs:		☐ STRENGTH	DURATION
	L	cal:	carbs:		☐ CARDIO	MILES
	D	cal:	carbs:			STEP COUNT
	S	cal:	carbs:		☐ FLEXIBILITY	CALORIES BURNT
WED	B	cal:	carbs:		☐ STRENGTH	DURATION
	L	cal:	carbs:		☐ CARDIO	MILES
	D	cal:	carbs:			STEP COUNT
	S	cal:	carbs:		☐ FLEXIBILITY	CALORIES BURNT
THUR	B	cal:	carbs:		☐ STRENGTH	DURATION
	L	cal:	carbs:		☐ CARDIO	MILES
	D	cal:	carbs:			STEP COUNT
	S	cal:	carbs:		☐ FLEXIBILITY	CALORIES BURNT
FRI	B	cal:	carbs:		☐ STRENGTH	DURATION
	L	cal:	carbs:		☐ CARDIO	MILES
	D	cal:	carbs:			STEP COUNT
	S	cal:	carbs:		☐ FLEXIBILITY	CALORIES BURNT
SAT	B	cal:	carbs:		☐ STRENGTH	DURATION
	L	cal:	carbs:		☐ CARDIO	MILES
	D	cal:	carbs:			STEP COUNT
	S	cal:	carbs:		☐ FLEXIBILITY	CALORIES BURNT

Health Tracker

	WEEKLY MEAL PLAN			WATER INTAKE	WORKOUT/EXERCISE	
SUN	B	cal:	carbs:		STRENGTH	DURATION
	L	cal:	carbs:			MILES
	D	cal:	carbs:		CARDIO	STEP COUNT
	S	cal:	carbs:		FLEXIBILITY	CALORIES BURNT
MON	B	cal:	carbs:		STRENGTH	DURATION
	L	cal:	carbs:			MILES
	D	cal:	carbs:		CARDIO	STEP COUNT
	S	cal:	carbs:		FLEXIBILITY	CALORIES BURNT
TUES	B	cal:	carbs:		STRENGTH	DURATION
	L	cal:	carbs:			MILES
	D	cal:	carbs:		CARDIO	STEP COUNT
	S	cal:	carbs:		FLEXIBILITY	CALORIES BURNT
WED	B	cal:	carbs:		STRENGTH	DURATION
	L	cal:	carbs:			MILES
	D	cal:	carbs:		CARDIO	STEP COUNT
	S	cal:	carbs:		FLEXIBILITY	CALORIES BURNT
THUR	B	cal:	carbs:		STRENGTH	DURATION
	L	cal:	carbs:			MILES
	D	cal:	carbs:		CARDIO	STEP COUNT
	S	cal:	carbs:		FLEXIBILITY	CALORIES BURNT
FRI	B	cal:	carbs:		STRENGTH	DURATION
	L	cal:	carbs:			MILES
	D	cal:	carbs:		CARDIO	STEP COUNT
	S	cal:	carbs:		FLEXIBILITY	CALORIES BURNT
SAT	B	cal:	carbs:		STRENGTH	DURATION
	L	cal:	carbs:			MILES
	D	cal:	carbs:		CARDIO	STEP COUNT
	S	cal:	carbs:		FLEXIBILITY	CALORIES BURNT

Health Tracker

	WEEKLY MEAL PLAN			WATER INTAKE	WORKOUT/EXERCISE	
SUN	B	cal:	carbs:		☐ STRENGTH	DURATION
	L	cal:	carbs:		☐ CARDIO	MILES
	D	cal:	carbs:			STEP COUNT
	S	cal:	carbs:		☐ FLEXIBILITY	CALORIES BURNT
MON	B	cal:	carbs:		☐ STRENGTH	DURATION
	L	cal:	carbs:		☐ CARDIO	MILES
	D	cal:	carbs:			STEP COUNT
	S	cal:	carbs:		☐ FLEXIBILITY	CALORIES BURNT
TUES	B	cal:	carbs:		☐ STRENGTH	DURATION
	L	cal:	carbs:		☐ CARDIO	MILES
	D	cal:	carbs:			STEP COUNT
	S	cal:	carbs:		☐ FLEXIBILITY	CALORIES BURNT
WED	B	cal:	carbs:		☐ STRENGTH	DURATION
	L	cal:	carbs:		☐ CARDIO	MILES
	D	cal:	carbs:			STEP COUNT
	S	cal:	carbs:		☐ FLEXIBILITY	CALORIES BURNT
THUR	B	cal:	carbs:		☐ STRENGTH	DURATION
	L	cal:	carbs:		☐ CARDIO	MILES
	D	cal:	carbs:			STEP COUNT
	S	cal:	carbs:		☐ FLEXIBILITY	CALORIES BURNT
FRI	B	cal:	carbs:		☐ STRENGTH	DURATION
	L	cal:	carbs:		☐ CARDIO	MILES
	D	cal:	carbs:			STEP COUNT
	S	cal:	carbs:		☐ FLEXIBILITY	CALORIES BURNT
SAT	B	cal:	carbs:		☐ STRENGTH	DURATION
	L	cal:	carbs:		☐ CARDIO	MILES
	D	cal:	carbs:			STEP COUNT
	S	cal:	carbs:		☐ FLEXIBILITY	CALORIES BURNT

Health Tracker

	WEEKLY MEAL PLAN			WATER INTAKE	WORKOUT/EXERCISE	
SUN	B	cal:	carbs:		STRENGTH	DURATION
	L	cal:	carbs:			MILES
	D	cal:	carbs:		CARDIO	STEP COUNT
	S	cal:	carbs:		FLEXIBILITY	CALORIES BURNT
MON	B	cal:	carbs:		STRENGTH	DURATION
	L	cal:	carbs:			MILES
	D	cal:	carbs:		CARDIO	STEP COUNT
	S	cal:	carbs:		FLEXIBILITY	CALORIES BURNT
TUES	B	cal:	carbs:		STRENGTH	DURATION
	L	cal:	carbs:			MILES
	D	cal:	carbs:		CARDIO	STEP COUNT
	S	cal:	carbs:		FLEXIBILITY	CALORIES BURNT
WED	B	cal:	carbs:		STRENGTH	DURATION
	L	cal:	carbs:			MILES
	D	cal:	carbs:		CARDIO	STEP COUNT
	S	cal:	carbs:		FLEXIBILITY	CALORIES BURNT
THUR	B	cal:	carbs:		STRENGTH	DURATION
	L	cal:	carbs:			MILES
	D	cal:	carbs:		CARDIO	STEP COUNT
	S	cal:	carbs:		FLEXIBILITY	CALORIES BURNT
FRI	B	cal:	carbs:		STRENGTH	DURATION
	L	cal:	carbs:			MILES
	D	cal:	carbs:		CARDIO	STEP COUNT
	S	cal:	carbs:		FLEXIBILITY	CALORIES BURNT
SAT	B	cal:	carbs:		STRENGTH	DURATION
	L	cal:	carbs:			MILES
	D	cal:	carbs:		CARDIO	STEP COUNT
	S	cal:	carbs:		FLEXIBILITY	CALORIES BURNT

WHAT'S ONE THING I'M DOING NOW THAT MY PAST SELF WOULD BE PROUD OF?

Health Tracker

	WEEKLY MEAL PLAN			WATER INTAKE	WORKOUT/EXERCISE	
SUN	B	cal:	carbs:		STRENGTH	DURATION
	L	cal:	carbs:		CARDIO	MILES
	D	cal:	carbs:			STEP COUNT
	S	cal:	carbs:		FLEXIBILITY	CALORIES BURNT
MON	B	cal:	carbs:		STRENGTH	DURATION
	L	cal:	carbs:		CARDIO	MILES
	D	cal:	carbs:			STEP COUNT
	S	cal:	carbs:		FLEXIBILITY	CALORIES BURNT
TUES	B	cal:	carbs:		STRENGTH	DURATION
	L	cal:	carbs:		CARDIO	MILES
	D	cal:	carbs:			STEP COUNT
	S	cal:	carbs:		FLEXIBILITY	CALORIES BURNT
WED	B	cal:	carbs:		STRENGTH	DURATION
	L	cal:	carbs:		CARDIO	MILES
	D	cal:	carbs:			STEP COUNT
	S	cal:	carbs:		FLEXIBILITY	CALORIES BURNT
THUR	B	cal:	carbs:		STRENGTH	DURATION
	L	cal:	carbs:		CARDIO	MILES
	D	cal:	carbs:			STEP COUNT
	S	cal:	carbs:		FLEXIBILITY	CALORIES BURNT
FRI	B	cal:	carbs:		STRENGTH	DURATION
	L	cal:	carbs:		CARDIO	MILES
	D	cal:	carbs:			STEP COUNT
	S	cal:	carbs:		FLEXIBILITY	CALORIES BURNT
SAT	B	cal:	carbs:		STRENGTH	DURATION
	L	cal:	carbs:		CARDIO	MILES
	D	cal:	carbs:			STEP COUNT
	S	cal:	carbs:		FLEXIBILITY	CALORIES BURNT

Health Tracker

	WEEKLY MEAL PLAN			WATER INTAKE	WORKOUT/EXERCISE	
SUN	B	cal:	carbs:		STRENGTH	DURATION
	L	cal:	carbs:			MILES
	D	cal:	carbs:		CARDIO	STEP COUNT
	S	cal:	carbs:		FLEXIBILITY	CALORIES BURNT
MON	B	cal:	carbs:		STRENGTH	DURATION
	L	cal:	carbs:			MILES
	D	cal:	carbs:		CARDIO	STEP COUNT
	S	cal:	carbs:		FLEXIBILITY	CALORIES BURNT
TUES	B	cal:	carbs:		STRENGTH	DURATION
	L	cal:	carbs:			MILES
	D	cal:	carbs:		CARDIO	STEP COUNT
	S	cal:	carbs:		FLEXIBILITY	CALORIES BURNT
WED	B	cal:	carbs:		STRENGTH	DURATION
	L	cal:	carbs:			MILES
	D	cal:	carbs:		CARDIO	STEP COUNT
	S	cal:	carbs:		FLEXIBILITY	CALORIES BURNT
THUR	B	cal:	carbs:		STRENGTH	DURATION
	L	cal:	carbs:			MILES
	D	cal:	carbs:		CARDIO	STEP COUNT
	S	cal:	carbs:		FLEXIBILITY	CALORIES BURNT
FRI	B	cal:	carbs:		STRENGTH	DURATION
	L	cal:	carbs:			MILES
	D	cal:	carbs:		CARDIO	STEP COUNT
	S	cal:	carbs:		FLEXIBILITY	CALORIES BURNT
SAT	B	cal:	carbs:		STRENGTH	DURATION
	L	cal:	carbs:			MILES
	D	cal:	carbs:		CARDIO	STEP COUNT
	S	cal:	carbs:		FLEXIBILITY	CALORIES BURNT

Health Tracker

	WEEKLY MEAL PLAN			WATER INTAKE	WORKOUT/EXERCISE	
SUN	B	cal:	carbs:		STRENGTH	DURATION
	L	cal:	carbs:		CARDIO	MILES
	D	cal:	carbs:			STEP COUNT
	S	cal:	carbs:		FLEXIBILITY	CALORIES BURNT
MON	B	cal:	carbs:		STRENGTH	DURATION
	L	cal:	carbs:		CARDIO	MILES
	D	cal:	carbs:			STEP COUNT
	S	cal:	carbs:		FLEXIBILITY	CALORIES BURNT
TUES	B	cal:	carbs:		STRENGTH	DURATION
	L	cal:	carbs:		CARDIO	MILES
	D	cal:	carbs:			STEP COUNT
	S	cal:	carbs:		FLEXIBILITY	CALORIES BURNT
WED	B	cal:	carbs:		STRENGTH	DURATION
	L	cal:	carbs:		CARDIO	MILES
	D	cal:	carbs:			STEP COUNT
	S	cal:	carbs:		FLEXIBILITY	CALORIES BURNT
THUR	B	cal:	carbs:		STRENGTH	DURATION
	L	cal:	carbs:		CARDIO	MILES
	D	cal:	carbs:			STEP COUNT
	S	cal:	carbs:		FLEXIBILITY	CALORIES BURNT
FRI	B	cal:	carbs:		STRENGTH	DURATION
	L	cal:	carbs:		CARDIO	MILES
	D	cal:	carbs:			STEP COUNT
	S	cal:	carbs:		FLEXIBILITY	CALORIES BURNT
SAT	B	cal:	carbs:		STRENGTH	DURATION
	L	cal:	carbs:		CARDIO	MILES
	D	cal:	carbs:			STEP COUNT
	S	cal:	carbs:		FLEXIBILITY	CALORIES BURNT

YOU WON'T
ALWAYS BE
MOTIVATED.
BE
DISCIPLINED
INSTEAD."

Health Tracker

WEEKLY MEAL PLAN			WATER INTAKE	WORKOUT/EXERCISE	
SUN					
B	cal:	carbs:		STRENGTH	DURATION
L	cal:	carbs:		CARDIO	MILES
D	cal:	carbs:			STEP COUNT
S	cal:	carbs:		FLEXIBILITY	CALORIES BURNT

WEEKLY MEAL PLAN			WATER INTAKE	WORKOUT/EXERCISE	
MON					
B	cal:	carbs:		STRENGTH	DURATION
L	cal:	carbs:		CARDIO	MILES
D	cal:	carbs:			STEP COUNT
S	cal:	carbs:		FLEXIBILITY	CALORIES BURNT

WEEKLY MEAL PLAN			WATER INTAKE	WORKOUT/EXERCISE	
TUES					
B	cal:	carbs:		STRENGTH	DURATION
L	cal:	carbs:		CARDIO	MILES
D	cal:	carbs:			STEP COUNT
S	cal:	carbs:		FLEXIBILITY	CALORIES BURNT

WEEKLY MEAL PLAN			WATER INTAKE	WORKOUT/EXERCISE	
WED					
B	cal:	carbs:		STRENGTH	DURATION
L	cal:	carbs:		CARDIO	MILES
D	cal:	carbs:			STEP COUNT
S	cal:	carbs:		FLEXIBILITY	CALORIES BURNT

WEEKLY MEAL PLAN			WATER INTAKE	WORKOUT/EXERCISE	
THUR					
B	cal:	carbs:		STRENGTH	DURATION
L	cal:	carbs:		CARDIO	MILES
D	cal:	carbs:			STEP COUNT
S	cal:	carbs:		FLEXIBILITY	CALORIES BURNT

WEEKLY MEAL PLAN			WATER INTAKE	WORKOUT/EXERCISE	
FRI					
B	cal:	carbs:		STRENGTH	DURATION
L	cal:	carbs:		CARDIO	MILES
D	cal:	carbs:			STEP COUNT
S	cal:	carbs:		FLEXIBILITY	CALORIES BURNT

WEEKLY MEAL PLAN			WATER INTAKE	WORKOUT/EXERCISE	
SAT					
B	cal:	carbs:		STRENGTH	DURATION
L	cal:	carbs:		CARDIO	MILES
D	cal:	carbs:			STEP COUNT
S	cal:	carbs:		FLEXIBILITY	CALORIES BURNT

Health Tracker

	WEEKLY MEAL PLAN			WATER INTAKE	WORKOUT/EXERCISE	
SUN	B	cal:	carbs:		STRENGTH	DURATION
	L	cal:	carbs:		CARDIO	MILES
	D	cal:	carbs:			STEP COUNT
	S	cal:	carbs:		FLEXIBILITY	CALORIES BURNT
MON	B	cal:	carbs:		STRENGTH	DURATION
	L	cal:	carbs:		CARDIO	MILES
	D	cal:	carbs:			STEP COUNT
	S	cal:	carbs:		FLEXIBILITY	CALORIES BURNT
TUES	B	cal:	carbs:		STRENGTH	DURATION
	L	cal:	carbs:		CARDIO	MILES
	D	cal:	carbs:			STEP COUNT
	S	cal:	carbs:		FLEXIBILITY	CALORIES BURNT
WED	B	cal:	carbs:		STRENGTH	DURATION
	L	cal:	carbs:		CARDIO	MILES
	D	cal:	carbs:			STEP COUNT
	S	cal:	carbs:		FLEXIBILITY	CALORIES BURNT
THUR	B	cal:	carbs:		STRENGTH	DURATION
	L	cal:	carbs:		CARDIO	MILES
	D	cal:	carbs:			STEP COUNT
	S	cal:	carbs:		FLEXIBILITY	CALORIES BURNT
FRI	B	cal:	carbs:		STRENGTH	DURATION
	L	cal:	carbs:		CARDIO	MILES
	D	cal:	carbs:			STEP COUNT
	S	cal:	carbs:		FLEXIBILITY	CALORIES BURNT
SAT	B	cal:	carbs:		STRENGTH	DURATION
	L	cal:	carbs:		CARDIO	MILES
	D	cal:	carbs:			STEP COUNT
	S	cal:	carbs:		FLEXIBILITY	CALORIES BURNT

Health Tracker

	WEEKLY MEAL PLAN			WATER INTAKE	WORKOUT/EXERCISE	
SUN	B	cal:	carbs:		☐ STRENGTH	DURATION
	L	cal:	carbs:		☐ CARDIO	MILES
	D	cal:	carbs:			STEP COUNT
	S	cal:	carbs:		☐ FLEXIBILITY	CALORIES BURNT
MON	B	cal:	carbs:		☐ STRENGTH	DURATION
	L	cal:	carbs:		☐ CARDIO	MILES
	D	cal:	carbs:			STEP COUNT
	S	cal:	carbs:		☐ FLEXIBILITY	CALORIES BURNT
TUES	B	cal:	carbs:		☐ STRENGTH	DURATION
	L	cal:	carbs:		☐ CARDIO	MILES
	D	cal:	carbs:			STEP COUNT
	S	cal:	carbs:		☐ FLEXIBILITY	CALORIES BURNT
WED	B	cal:	carbs:		☐ STRENGTH	DURATION
	L	cal:	carbs:		☐ CARDIO	MILES
	D	cal:	carbs:			STEP COUNT
	S	cal:	carbs:		☐ FLEXIBILITY	CALORIES BURNT
THUR	B	cal:	carbs:		☐ STRENGTH	DURATION
	L	cal:	carbs:		☐ CARDIO	MILES
	D	cal:	carbs:			STEP COUNT
	S	cal:	carbs:		☐ FLEXIBILITY	CALORIES BURNT
FRI	B	cal:	carbs:		☐ STRENGTH	DURATION
	L	cal:	carbs:		☐ CARDIO	MILES
	D	cal:	carbs:			STEP COUNT
	S	cal:	carbs:		☐ FLEXIBILITY	CALORIES BURNT
SAT	B	cal:	carbs:		☐ STRENGTH	DURATION
	L	cal:	carbs:		☐ CARDIO	MILES
	D	cal:	carbs:			STEP COUNT
	S	cal:	carbs:		☐ FLEXIBILITY	CALORIES BURNT

Health Tracker

	WEEKLY MEAL PLAN			WATER INTAKE	WORKOUT/EXERCISE	
SUN	B	cal:	carbs:		☐ STRENGTH	DURATION
	L	cal:	carbs:		☐ CARDIO	MILES
	D	cal:	carbs:			STEP COUNT
	S	cal:	carbs:		☐ FLEXIBILITY	CALORIES BURNT
MON	B	cal:	carbs:		☐ STRENGTH	DURATION
	L	cal:	carbs:		☐ CARDIO	MILES
	D	cal:	carbs:			STEP COUNT
	S	cal:	carbs:		☐ FLEXIBILITY	CALORIES BURNT
TUES	B	cal:	carbs:		☐ STRENGTH	DURATION
	L	cal:	carbs:		☐ CARDIO	MILES
	D	cal:	carbs:			STEP COUNT
	S	cal:	carbs:		☐ FLEXIBILITY	CALORIES BURNT
WED	B	cal:	carbs:		☐ STRENGTH	DURATION
	L	cal:	carbs:		☐ CARDIO	MILES
	D	cal:	carbs:			STEP COUNT
	S	cal:	carbs:		☐ FLEXIBILITY	CALORIES BURNT
THUR	B	cal:	carbs:		☐ STRENGTH	DURATION
	L	cal:	carbs:		☐ CARDIO	MILES
	D	cal:	carbs:			STEP COUNT
	S	cal:	carbs:		☐ FLEXIBILITY	CALORIES BURNT
FRI	B	cal:	carbs:		☐ STRENGTH	DURATION
	L	cal:	carbs:		☐ CARDIO	MILES
	D	cal:	carbs:			STEP COUNT
	S	cal:	carbs:		☐ FLEXIBILITY	CALORIES BURNT
SAT	B	cal:	carbs:		☐ STRENGTH	DURATION
	L	cal:	carbs:		☐ CARDIO	MILES
	D	cal:	carbs:			STEP COUNT
	S	cal:	carbs:		☐ FLEXIBILITY	CALORIES BURNT

WHERE DID I SHOW UP WHEN IT WAS HARDEST?

Health Tracker

	WEEKLY MEAL PLAN			WATER INTAKE	WORKOUT/EXERCISE	
SUN	B	cal:	carbs:		☐ STRENGTH	DURATION
	L	cal:	carbs:		☐ CARDIO	MILES
	D	cal:	carbs:			STEP COUNT
	S	cal:	carbs:		☐ FLEXIBILITY	CALORIES BURNT
MON	B	cal:	carbs:		☐ STRENGTH	DURATION
	L	cal:	carbs:		☐ CARDIO	MILES
	D	cal:	carbs:			STEP COUNT
	S	cal:	carbs:		☐ FLEXIBILITY	CALORIES BURNT
TUES	B	cal:	carbs:		☐ STRENGTH	DURATION
	L	cal:	carbs:		☐ CARDIO	MILES
	D	cal:	carbs:			STEP COUNT
	S	cal:	carbs:		☐ FLEXIBILITY	CALORIES BURNT
WED	B	cal:	carbs:		☐ STRENGTH	DURATION
	L	cal:	carbs:		☐ CARDIO	MILES
	D	cal:	carbs:			STEP COUNT
	S	cal:	carbs:		☐ FLEXIBILITY	CALORIES BURNT
THUR	B	cal:	carbs:		☐ STRENGTH	DURATION
	L	cal:	carbs:		☐ CARDIO	MILES
	D	cal:	carbs:			STEP COUNT
	S	cal:	carbs:		☐ FLEXIBILITY	CALORIES BURNT
FRI	B	cal:	carbs:		☐ STRENGTH	DURATION
	L	cal:	carbs:		☐ CARDIO	MILES
	D	cal:	carbs:			STEP COUNT
	S	cal:	carbs:		☐ FLEXIBILITY	CALORIES BURNT
SAT	B	cal:	carbs:		☐ STRENGTH	DURATION
	L	cal:	carbs:		☐ CARDIO	MILES
	D	cal:	carbs:			STEP COUNT
	S	cal:	carbs:		☐ FLEXIBILITY	CALORIES BURNT

Health Tracker

	WEEKLY MEAL PLAN			WATER INTAKE	WORKOUT/EXERCISE	
SUN	B	cal:	carbs:		STRENGTH	DURATION
	L	cal:	carbs:		CARDIO	MILES
	D	cal:	carbs:			STEP COUNT
	S	cal:	carbs:		FLEXIBILITY	CALORIES BURNT
MON	B	cal:	carbs:		STRENGTH	DURATION
	L	cal:	carbs:		CARDIO	MILES
	D	cal:	carbs:			STEP COUNT
	S	cal:	carbs:		FLEXIBILITY	CALORIES BURNT
TUES	B	cal:	carbs:		STRENGTH	DURATION
	L	cal:	carbs:		CARDIO	MILES
	D	cal:	carbs:			STEP COUNT
	S	cal:	carbs:		FLEXIBILITY	CALORIES BURNT
WED	B	cal:	carbs:		STRENGTH	DURATION
	L	cal:	carbs:		CARDIO	MILES
	D	cal:	carbs:			STEP COUNT
	S	cal:	carbs:		FLEXIBILITY	CALORIES BURNT
THUR	B	cal:	carbs:		STRENGTH	DURATION
	L	cal:	carbs:		CARDIO	MILES
	D	cal:	carbs:			STEP COUNT
	S	cal:	carbs:		FLEXIBILITY	CALORIES BURNT
FRI	B	cal:	carbs:		STRENGTH	DURATION
	L	cal:	carbs:		CARDIO	MILES
	D	cal:	carbs:			STEP COUNT
	S	cal:	carbs:		FLEXIBILITY	CALORIES BURNT
SAT	B	cal:	carbs:		STRENGTH	DURATION
	L	cal:	carbs:		CARDIO	MILES
	D	cal:	carbs:			STEP COUNT
	S	cal:	carbs:		FLEXIBILITY	CALORIES BURNT

Health Tracker

	WEEKLY MEAL PLAN			WATER INTAKE	WORKOUT/EXERCISE	
SUN	B	cal:	carbs:		STRENGTH	DURATION
	L	cal:	carbs:		CARDIO	MILES
	D	cal:	carbs:			STEP COUNT
	S	cal:	carbs:		FLEXIBILITY	CALORIES BURNT
MON	B	cal:	carbs:		STRENGTH	DURATION
	L	cal:	carbs:		CARDIO	MILES
	D	cal:	carbs:			STEP COUNT
	S	cal:	carbs:		FLEXIBILITY	CALORIES BURNT
TUES	B	cal:	carbs:		STRENGTH	DURATION
	L	cal:	carbs:		CARDIO	MILES
	D	cal:	carbs:			STEP COUNT
	S	cal:	carbs:		FLEXIBILITY	CALORIES BURNT
WED	B	cal:	carbs:		STRENGTH	DURATION
	L	cal:	carbs:		CARDIO	MILES
	D	cal:	carbs:			STEP COUNT
	S	cal:	carbs:		FLEXIBILITY	CALORIES BURNT
THUR	B	cal:	carbs:		STRENGTH	DURATION
	L	cal:	carbs:		CARDIO	MILES
	D	cal:	carbs:			STEP COUNT
	S	cal:	carbs:		FLEXIBILITY	CALORIES BURNT
FRI	B	cal:	carbs:		STRENGTH	DURATION
	L	cal:	carbs:		CARDIO	MILES
	D	cal:	carbs:			STEP COUNT
	S	cal:	carbs:		FLEXIBILITY	CALORIES BURNT
SAT	B	cal:	carbs:		STRENGTH	DURATION
	L	cal:	carbs:		CARDIO	MILES
	D	cal:	carbs:			STEP COUNT
	S	cal:	carbs:		FLEXIBILITY	CALORIES BURNT

Health Tracker

	WEEKLY MEAL PLAN			WATER INTAKE	WORKOUT/EXERCISE	
SUN	B	cal:	carbs:		STRENGTH	DURATION
	L	cal:	carbs:		CARDIO	MILES
	D	cal:	carbs:			STEP COUNT
	S	cal:	carbs:		FLEXIBILITY	CALORIES BURNT
MON	B	cal:	carbs:		STRENGTH	DURATION
	L	cal:	carbs:		CARDIO	MILES
	D	cal:	carbs:			STEP COUNT
	S	cal:	carbs:		FLEXIBILITY	CALORIES BURNT
TUES	B	cal:	carbs:		STRENGTH	DURATION
	L	cal:	carbs:		CARDIO	MILES
	D	cal:	carbs:			STEP COUNT
	S	cal:	carbs:		FLEXIBILITY	CALORIES BURNT
WED	B	cal:	carbs:		STRENGTH	DURATION
	L	cal:	carbs:		CARDIO	MILES
	D	cal:	carbs:			STEP COUNT
	S	cal:	carbs:		FLEXIBILITY	CALORIES BURNT
THUR	B	cal:	carbs:		STRENGTH	DURATION
	L	cal:	carbs:		CARDIO	MILES
	D	cal:	carbs:			STEP COUNT
	S	cal:	carbs:		FLEXIBILITY	CALORIES BURNT
FRI	B	cal:	carbs:		STRENGTH	DURATION
	L	cal:	carbs:		CARDIO	MILES
	D	cal:	carbs:			STEP COUNT
	S	cal:	carbs:		FLEXIBILITY	CALORIES BURNT
SAT	B	cal:	carbs:		STRENGTH	DURATION
	L	cal:	carbs:		CARDIO	MILES
	D	cal:	carbs:			STEP COUNT
	S	cal:	carbs:		FLEXIBILITY	CALORIES BURNT

"EVERY DROP OF SWEAT IS A RECEIPT."

Health Tracker

	WEEKLY MEAL PLAN			WATER INTAKE	WORKOUT/EXERCISE	
SUN	B	cal:	carbs:		STRENGTH	DURATION
	L	cal:	carbs:		CARDIO	MILES
	D	cal:	carbs:			STEP COUNT
	S	cal:	carbs:		FLEXIBILITY	CALORIES BURNT
MON	B	cal:	carbs:		STRENGTH	DURATION
	L	cal:	carbs:		CARDIO	MILES
	D	cal:	carbs:			STEP COUNT
	S	cal:	carbs:		FLEXIBILITY	CALORIES BURNT
TUES	B	cal:	carbs:		STRENGTH	DURATION
	L	cal:	carbs:		CARDIO	MILES
	D	cal:	carbs:			STEP COUNT
	S	cal:	carbs:		FLEXIBILITY	CALORIES BURNT
WED	B	cal:	carbs:		STRENGTH	DURATION
	L	cal:	carbs:		CARDIO	MILES
	D	cal:	carbs:			STEP COUNT
	S	cal:	carbs:		FLEXIBILITY	CALORIES BURNT
THUR	B	cal:	carbs:		STRENGTH	DURATION
	L	cal:	carbs:		CARDIO	MILES
	D	cal:	carbs:			STEP COUNT
	S	cal:	carbs:		FLEXIBILITY	CALORIES BURNT
FRI	B	cal:	carbs:		STRENGTH	DURATION
	L	cal:	carbs:		CARDIO	MILES
	D	cal:	carbs:			STEP COUNT
	S	cal:	carbs:		FLEXIBILITY	CALORIES BURNT
SAT	B	cal:	carbs:		STRENGTH	DURATION
	L	cal:	carbs:		CARDIO	MILES
	D	cal:	carbs:			STEP COUNT
	S	cal:	carbs:		FLEXIBILITY	CALORIES BURNT

Health Tracker

	WEEKLY MEAL PLAN			WATER INTAKE	WORKOUT/EXERCISE	
SUN	B	cal:	carbs:		STRENGTH	DURATION
	L	cal:	carbs:		CARDIO	MILES
	D	cal:	carbs:			STEP COUNT
	S	cal:	carbs:		FLEXIBILITY	CALORIES BURNT
MON	B	cal:	carbs:		STRENGTH	DURATION
	L	cal:	carbs:		CARDIO	MILES
	D	cal:	carbs:			STEP COUNT
	S	cal:	carbs:		FLEXIBILITY	CALORIES BURNT
TUES	B	cal:	carbs:		STRENGTH	DURATION
	L	cal:	carbs:		CARDIO	MILES
	D	cal:	carbs:			STEP COUNT
	S	cal:	carbs:		FLEXIBILITY	CALORIES BURNT
WED	B	cal:	carbs:		STRENGTH	DURATION
	L	cal:	carbs:		CARDIO	MILES
	D	cal:	carbs:			STEP COUNT
	S	cal:	carbs:		FLEXIBILITY	CALORIES BURNT
THUR	B	cal:	carbs:		STRENGTH	DURATION
	L	cal:	carbs:		CARDIO	MILES
	D	cal:	carbs:			STEP COUNT
	S	cal:	carbs:		FLEXIBILITY	CALORIES BURNT
FRI	B	cal:	carbs:		STRENGTH	DURATION
	L	cal:	carbs:		CARDIO	MILES
	D	cal:	carbs:			STEP COUNT
	S	cal:	carbs:		FLEXIBILITY	CALORIES BURNT
SAT	B	cal:	carbs:		STRENGTH	DURATION
	L	cal:	carbs:		CARDIO	MILES
	D	cal:	carbs:			STEP COUNT
	S	cal:	carbs:		FLEXIBILITY	CALORIES BURNT

Health Tracker ____________________

	WEEKLY MEAL PLAN			WATER INTAKE	WORKOUT/EXERCISE	
SUN	B	cal:	carbs:		STRENGTH	DURATION
	L	cal:	carbs:		CARDIO	MILES
	D	cal:	carbs:			STEP COUNT
	S	cal:	carbs:		FLEXIBILITY	CALORIES BURNT
MON	B	cal:	carbs:		STRENGTH	DURATION
	L	cal:	carbs:		CARDIO	MILES
	D	cal:	carbs:			STEP COUNT
	S	cal:	carbs:		FLEXIBILITY	CALORIES BURNT
TUES	B	cal:	carbs:		STRENGTH	DURATION
	L	cal:	carbs:		CARDIO	MILES
	D	cal:	carbs:			STEP COUNT
	S	cal:	carbs:		FLEXIBILITY	CALORIES BURNT
WED	B	cal:	carbs:		STRENGTH	DURATION
	L	cal:	carbs:		CARDIO	MILES
	D	cal:	carbs:			STEP COUNT
	S	cal:	carbs:		FLEXIBILITY	CALORIES BURNT
THUR	B	cal:	carbs:		STRENGTH	DURATION
	L	cal:	carbs:		CARDIO	MILES
	D	cal:	carbs:			STEP COUNT
	S	cal:	carbs:		FLEXIBILITY	CALORIES BURNT
FRI	B	cal:	carbs:		STRENGTH	DURATION
	L	cal:	carbs:		CARDIO	MILES
	D	cal:	carbs:			STEP COUNT
	S	cal:	carbs:		FLEXIBILITY	CALORIES BURNT
SAT	B	cal:	carbs:		STRENGTH	DURATION
	L	cal:	carbs:		CARDIO	MILES
	D	cal:	carbs:			STEP COUNT
	S	cal:	carbs:		FLEXIBILITY	CALORIES BURNT

Health Tracker

Day	WEEKLY MEAL PLAN			WATER INTAKE	WORKOUT/EXERCISE	
SUN	B	cal:	carbs:		STRENGTH	DURATION
	L	cal:	carbs:			MILES
	D	cal:	carbs:		CARDIO	STEP COUNT
	S	cal:	carbs:		FLEXIBILITY	CALORIES BURNT
MON	B	cal:	carbs:		STRENGTH	DURATION
	L	cal:	carbs:			MILES
	D	cal:	carbs:		CARDIO	STEP COUNT
	S	cal:	carbs:		FLEXIBILITY	CALORIES BURNT
TUES	B	cal:	carbs:		STRENGTH	DURATION
	L	cal:	carbs:			MILES
	D	cal:	carbs:		CARDIO	STEP COUNT
	S	cal:	carbs:		FLEXIBILITY	CALORIES BURNT
WED	B	cal:	carbs:		STRENGTH	DURATION
	L	cal:	carbs:			MILES
	D	cal:	carbs:		CARDIO	STEP COUNT
	S	cal:	carbs:		FLEXIBILITY	CALORIES BURNT
THUR	B	cal:	carbs:		STRENGTH	DURATION
	L	cal:	carbs:			MILES
	D	cal:	carbs:		CARDIO	STEP COUNT
	S	cal:	carbs:		FLEXIBILITY	CALORIES BURNT
FRI	B	cal:	carbs:		STRENGTH	DURATION
	L	cal:	carbs:			MILES
	D	cal:	carbs:		CARDIO	STEP COUNT
	S	cal:	carbs:		FLEXIBILITY	CALORIES BURNT
SAT	B	cal:	carbs:		STRENGTH	DURATION
	L	cal:	carbs:			MILES
	D	cal:	carbs:		CARDIO	STEP COUNT
	S	cal:	carbs:		FLEXIBILITY	CALORIES BURNT

WHAT EXCUSE DID I SILENCE AND HOW?

Health Tracker

	WEEKLY MEAL PLAN			WATER INTAKE	WORKOUT/EXERCISE	
SUN	B	cal:	carbs:		STRENGTH	DURATION
	L	cal:	carbs:		CARDIO	MILES
	D	cal:	carbs:			STEP COUNT
	S	cal:	carbs:		FLEXIBILITY	CALORIES BURNT
MON	B	cal:	carbs:		STRENGTH	DURATION
	L	cal:	carbs:		CARDIO	MILES
	D	cal:	carbs:			STEP COUNT
	S	cal:	carbs:		FLEXIBILITY	CALORIES BURNT
TUES	B	cal:	carbs:		STRENGTH	DURATION
	L	cal:	carbs:		CARDIO	MILES
	D	cal:	carbs:			STEP COUNT
	S	cal:	carbs:		FLEXIBILITY	CALORIES BURNT
WED	B	cal:	carbs:		STRENGTH	DURATION
	L	cal:	carbs:		CARDIO	MILES
	D	cal:	carbs:			STEP COUNT
	S	cal:	carbs:		FLEXIBILITY	CALORIES BURNT
THUR	B	cal:	carbs:		STRENGTH	DURATION
	L	cal:	carbs:		CARDIO	MILES
	D	cal:	carbs:			STEP COUNT
	S	cal:	carbs:		FLEXIBILITY	CALORIES BURNT
FRI	B	cal:	carbs:		STRENGTH	DURATION
	L	cal:	carbs:		CARDIO	MILES
	D	cal:	carbs:			STEP COUNT
	S	cal:	carbs:		FLEXIBILITY	CALORIES BURNT
SAT	B	cal:	carbs:		STRENGTH	DURATION
	L	cal:	carbs:		CARDIO	MILES
	D	cal:	carbs:			STEP COUNT
	S	cal:	carbs:		FLEXIBILITY	CALORIES BURNT

Health Tracker

	WEEKLY MEAL PLAN			WATER INTAKE	WORKOUT/EXERCISE	
SUN	B	cal:	carbs:		☐ STRENGTH	DURATION
	L	cal:	carbs:		☐ CARDIO	MILES
	D	cal:	carbs:			STEP COUNT
	S	cal:	carbs:		☐ FLEXIBILITY	CALORIES BURNT
MON	B	cal:	carbs:		☐ STRENGTH	DURATION
	L	cal:	carbs:		☐ CARDIO	MILES
	D	cal:	carbs:			STEP COUNT
	S	cal:	carbs:		☐ FLEXIBILITY	CALORIES BURNT
TUES	B	cal:	carbs:		☐ STRENGTH	DURATION
	L	cal:	carbs:		☐ CARDIO	MILES
	D	cal:	carbs:			STEP COUNT
	S	cal:	carbs:		☐ FLEXIBILITY	CALORIES BURNT
WED	B	cal:	carbs:		☐ STRENGTH	DURATION
	L	cal:	carbs:		☐ CARDIO	MILES
	D	cal:	carbs:			STEP COUNT
	S	cal:	carbs:		☐ FLEXIBILITY	CALORIES BURNT
THUR	B	cal:	carbs:		☐ STRENGTH	DURATION
	L	cal:	carbs:		☐ CARDIO	MILES
	D	cal:	carbs:			STEP COUNT
	S	cal:	carbs:		☐ FLEXIBILITY	CALORIES BURNT
FRI	B	cal:	carbs:		☐ STRENGTH	DURATION
	L	cal:	carbs:		☐ CARDIO	MILES
	D	cal:	carbs:			STEP COUNT
	S	cal:	carbs:		☐ FLEXIBILITY	CALORIES BURNT
SAT	B	cal:	carbs:		☐ STRENGTH	DURATION
	L	cal:	carbs:		☐ CARDIO	MILES
	D	cal:	carbs:			STEP COUNT
	S	cal:	carbs:		☐ FLEXIBILITY	CALORIES BURNT

Health Tracker

	WEEKLY MEAL PLAN			WATER INTAKE	WORKOUT/EXERCISE	
SUN	B	cal:	carbs:		STRENGTH	DURATION
	L	cal:	carbs:		CARDIO	MILES
	D	cal:	carbs:			STEP COUNT
	S	cal:	carbs:		FLEXIBILITY	CALORIES BURNT
MON	B	cal:	carbs:		STRENGTH	DURATION
	L	cal:	carbs:		CARDIO	MILES
	D	cal:	carbs:			STEP COUNT
	S	cal:	carbs:		FLEXIBILITY	CALORIES BURNT
TUES	B	cal:	carbs:		STRENGTH	DURATION
	L	cal:	carbs:		CARDIO	MILES
	D	cal:	carbs:			STEP COUNT
	S	cal:	carbs:		FLEXIBILITY	CALORIES BURNT
WED	B	cal:	carbs:		STRENGTH	DURATION
	L	cal:	carbs:		CARDIO	MILES
	D	cal:	carbs:			STEP COUNT
	S	cal:	carbs:		FLEXIBILITY	CALORIES BURNT
THUR	B	cal:	carbs:		STRENGTH	DURATION
	L	cal:	carbs:		CARDIO	MILES
	D	cal:	carbs:			STEP COUNT
	S	cal:	carbs:		FLEXIBILITY	CALORIES BURNT
FRI	B	cal:	carbs:		STRENGTH	DURATION
	L	cal:	carbs:		CARDIO	MILES
	D	cal:	carbs:			STEP COUNT
	S	cal:	carbs:		FLEXIBILITY	CALORIES BURNT
SAT	B	cal:	carbs:		STRENGTH	DURATION
	L	cal:	carbs:		CARDIO	MILES
	D	cal:	carbs:			STEP COUNT
	S	cal:	carbs:		FLEXIBILITY	CALORIES BURNT

Health Tracker

	WEEKLY MEAL PLAN			WATER INTAKE	WORKOUT/EXERCISE	
SUN	B	cal:	carbs:		STRENGTH	DURATION
	L	cal:	carbs:			MILES
	D	cal:	carbs:		CARDIO	STEP COUNT
	S	cal:	carbs:		FLEXIBILITY	CALORIES BURNT

MON	B	cal:	carbs:		STRENGTH	DURATION
	L	cal:	carbs:			MILES
	D	cal:	carbs:		CARDIO	STEP COUNT
	S	cal:	carbs:		FLEXIBILITY	CALORIES BURNT

TUES	B	cal:	carbs:		STRENGTH	DURATION
	L	cal:	carbs:			MILES
	D	cal:	carbs:		CARDIO	STEP COUNT
	S	cal:	carbs:		FLEXIBILITY	CALORIES BURNT

WED	B	cal:	carbs:		STRENGTH	DURATION
	L	cal:	carbs:			MILES
	D	cal:	carbs:		CARDIO	STEP COUNT
	S	cal:	carbs:		FLEXIBILITY	CALORIES BURNT

THUR	B	cal:	carbs:		STRENGTH	DURATION
	L	cal:	carbs:			MILES
	D	cal:	carbs:		CARDIO	STEP COUNT
	S	cal:	carbs:		FLEXIBILITY	CALORIES BURNT

FRI	B	cal:	carbs:		STRENGTH	DURATION
	L	cal:	carbs:			MILES
	D	cal:	carbs:		CARDIO	STEP COUNT
	S	cal:	carbs:		FLEXIBILITY	CALORIES BURNT

SAT	B	cal:	carbs:		STRENGTH	DURATION
	L	cal:	carbs:			MILES
	D	cal:	carbs:		CARDIO	STEP COUNT
	S	cal:	carbs:		FLEXIBILITY	CALORIES BURNT

WHAT DID I PUSH THROUGH THIS WEEK THAT I WOULD'VE QUIT BEFORE?

Health Tracker

	WEEKLY MEAL PLAN			WATER INTAKE	WORKOUT/EXERCISE	
SUN	B	cal:	carbs:		☐ STRENGTH	DURATION
	L	cal:	carbs:			MILES
	D	cal:	carbs:		☐ CARDIO	STEP COUNT
	S	cal:	carbs:		☐ FLEXIBILITY	CALORIES BURNT
MON	B	cal:	carbs:		☐ STRENGTH	DURATION
	L	cal:	carbs:			MILES
	D	cal:	carbs:		☐ CARDIO	STEP COUNT
	S	cal:	carbs:		☐ FLEXIBILITY	CALORIES BURNT
TUES	B	cal:	carbs:		☐ STRENGTH	DURATION
	L	cal:	carbs:			MILES
	D	cal:	carbs:		☐ CARDIO	STEP COUNT
	S	cal:	carbs:		☐ FLEXIBILITY	CALORIES BURNT
WED	B	cal:	carbs:		☐ STRENGTH	DURATION
	L	cal:	carbs:			MILES
	D	cal:	carbs:		☐ CARDIO	STEP COUNT
	S	cal:	carbs:		☐ FLEXIBILITY	CALORIES BURNT
THUR	B	cal:	carbs:		☐ STRENGTH	DURATION
	L	cal:	carbs:			MILES
	D	cal:	carbs:		☐ CARDIO	STEP COUNT
	S	cal:	carbs:		☐ FLEXIBILITY	CALORIES BURNT
FRI	B	cal:	carbs:		☐ STRENGTH	DURATION
	L	cal:	carbs:			MILES
	D	cal:	carbs:		☐ CARDIO	STEP COUNT
	S	cal:	carbs:		☐ FLEXIBILITY	CALORIES BURNT
SAT	B	cal:	carbs:		☐ STRENGTH	DURATION
	L	cal:	carbs:			MILES
	D	cal:	carbs:		☐ CARDIO	STEP COUNT
	S	cal:	carbs:		☐ FLEXIBILITY	CALORIES BURNT

"THEY'LL SEE RESULTS. YOU'LL FEEL THEM."

Health Tracker

	WEEKLY MEAL PLAN			WATER INTAKE	WORKOUT/EXERCISE	
SUN	B	cal:	carbs:		STRENGTH	DURATION
	L	cal:	carbs:		CARDIO	MILES
	D	cal:	carbs:			STEP COUNT
	S	cal:	carbs:		FLEXIBILITY	CALORIES BURNT
MON	B	cal:	carbs:		STRENGTH	DURATION
	L	cal:	carbs:		CARDIO	MILES
	D	cal:	carbs:			STEP COUNT
	S	cal:	carbs:		FLEXIBILITY	CALORIES BURNT
TUES	B	cal:	carbs:		STRENGTH	DURATION
	L	cal:	carbs:		CARDIO	MILES
	D	cal:	carbs:			STEP COUNT
	S	cal:	carbs:		FLEXIBILITY	CALORIES BURNT
WED	B	cal:	carbs:		STRENGTH	DURATION
	L	cal:	carbs:		CARDIO	MILES
	D	cal:	carbs:			STEP COUNT
	S	cal:	carbs:		FLEXIBILITY	CALORIES BURNT
THUR	B	cal:	carbs:		STRENGTH	DURATION
	L	cal:	carbs:		CARDIO	MILES
	D	cal:	carbs:			STEP COUNT
	S	cal:	carbs:		FLEXIBILITY	CALORIES BURNT
FRI	B	cal:	carbs:		STRENGTH	DURATION
	L	cal:	carbs:		CARDIO	MILES
	D	cal:	carbs:			STEP COUNT
	S	cal:	carbs:		FLEXIBILITY	CALORIES BURNT
SAT	B	cal:	carbs:		STRENGTH	DURATION
	L	cal:	carbs:		CARDIO	MILES
	D	cal:	carbs:			STEP COUNT
	S	cal:	carbs:		FLEXIBILITY	CALORIES BURNT

Health Tracker

	WEEKLY MEAL PLAN			WATER INTAKE	WORKOUT/EXERCISE	
SUN	B	cal:	carbs:		☐ STRENGTH	DURATION
	L	cal:	carbs:		☐ CARDIO	MILES
	D	cal:	carbs:			STEP COUNT
	S	cal:	carbs:		☐ FLEXIBILITY	CALORIES BURNT
MON	B	cal:	carbs:		☐ STRENGTH	DURATION
	L	cal:	carbs:		☐ CARDIO	MILES
	D	cal:	carbs:			STEP COUNT
	S	cal:	carbs:		☐ FLEXIBILITY	CALORIES BURNT
TUES	B	cal:	carbs:		☐ STRENGTH	DURATION
	L	cal:	carbs:		☐ CARDIO	MILES
	D	cal:	carbs:			STEP COUNT
	S	cal:	carbs:		☐ FLEXIBILITY	CALORIES BURNT
WED	B	cal:	carbs:		☐ STRENGTH	DURATION
	L	cal:	carbs:		☐ CARDIO	MILES
	D	cal:	carbs:			STEP COUNT
	S	cal:	carbs:		☐ FLEXIBILITY	CALORIES BURNT
THUR	B	cal:	carbs:		☐ STRENGTH	DURATION
	L	cal:	carbs:		☐ CARDIO	MILES
	D	cal:	carbs:			STEP COUNT
	S	cal:	carbs:		☐ FLEXIBILITY	CALORIES BURNT
FRI	B	cal:	carbs:		☐ STRENGTH	DURATION
	L	cal:	carbs:		☐ CARDIO	MILES
	D	cal:	carbs:			STEP COUNT
	S	cal:	carbs:		☐ FLEXIBILITY	CALORIES BURNT
SAT	B	cal:	carbs:		☐ STRENGTH	DURATION
	L	cal:	carbs:		☐ CARDIO	MILES
	D	cal:	carbs:			STEP COUNT
	S	cal:	carbs:		☐ FLEXIBILITY	CALORIES BURNT

Health Tracker

	WEEKLY MEAL PLAN			WATER INTAKE	WORKOUT/EXERCISE	
SUN	B	cal:	carbs:		STRENGTH	DURATION
	L	cal:	carbs:		CARDIO	MILES
	D	cal:	carbs:			STEP COUNT
	S	cal:	carbs:		FLEXIBILITY	CALORIES BURNT
MON	B	cal:	carbs:		STRENGTH	DURATION
	L	cal:	carbs:		CARDIO	MILES
	D	cal:	carbs:			STEP COUNT
	S	cal:	carbs:		FLEXIBILITY	CALORIES BURNT
TUES	B	cal:	carbs:		STRENGTH	DURATION
	L	cal:	carbs:		CARDIO	MILES
	D	cal:	carbs:			STEP COUNT
	S	cal:	carbs:		FLEXIBILITY	CALORIES BURNT
WED	B	cal:	carbs:		STRENGTH	DURATION
	L	cal:	carbs:		CARDIO	MILES
	D	cal:	carbs:			STEP COUNT
	S	cal:	carbs:		FLEXIBILITY	CALORIES BURNT
THUR	B	cal:	carbs:		STRENGTH	DURATION
	L	cal:	carbs:		CARDIO	MILES
	D	cal:	carbs:			STEP COUNT
	S	cal:	carbs:		FLEXIBILITY	CALORIES BURNT
FRI	B	cal:	carbs:		STRENGTH	DURATION
	L	cal:	carbs:		CARDIO	MILES
	D	cal:	carbs:			STEP COUNT
	S	cal:	carbs:		FLEXIBILITY	CALORIES BURNT
SAT	B	cal:	carbs:		STRENGTH	DURATION
	L	cal:	carbs:		CARDIO	MILES
	D	cal:	carbs:			STEP COUNT
	S	cal:	carbs:		FLEXIBILITY	CALORIES BURNT

Health Tracker

	WEEKLY MEAL PLAN			WATER INTAKE	WORKOUT/EXERCISE	
SUN	B	cal:	carbs:		STRENGTH	DURATION
	L	cal:	carbs:		CARDIO	MILES
	D	cal:	carbs:			STEP COUNT
	S	cal:	carbs:		FLEXIBILITY	CALORIES BURNT
MON	B	cal:	carbs:		STRENGTH	DURATION
	L	cal:	carbs:		CARDIO	MILES
	D	cal:	carbs:			STEP COUNT
	S	cal:	carbs:		FLEXIBILITY	CALORIES BURNT
TUES	B	cal:	carbs:		STRENGTH	DURATION
	L	cal:	carbs:		CARDIO	MILES
	D	cal:	carbs:			STEP COUNT
	S	cal:	carbs:		FLEXIBILITY	CALORIES BURNT
WED	B	cal:	carbs:		STRENGTH	DURATION
	L	cal:	carbs:		CARDIO	MILES
	D	cal:	carbs:			STEP COUNT
	S	cal:	carbs:		FLEXIBILITY	CALORIES BURNT
THUR	B	cal:	carbs:		STRENGTH	DURATION
	L	cal:	carbs:		CARDIO	MILES
	D	cal:	carbs:			STEP COUNT
	S	cal:	carbs:		FLEXIBILITY	CALORIES BURNT
FRI	B	cal:	carbs:		STRENGTH	DURATION
	L	cal:	carbs:		CARDIO	MILES
	D	cal:	carbs:			STEP COUNT
	S	cal:	carbs:		FLEXIBILITY	CALORIES BURNT
SAT	B	cal:	carbs:		STRENGTH	DURATION
	L	cal:	carbs:		CARDIO	MILES
	D	cal:	carbs:			STEP COUNT
	S	cal:	carbs:		FLEXIBILITY	CALORIES BURNT

"PROVE TO YOURSELF THAT YOU CAN DO HARD THINGS."

Health Tracker

	WEEKLY MEAL PLAN			WATER INTAKE	WORKOUT/EXERCISE	
SUN	B	cal:	carbs:		STRENGTH	DURATION
	L	cal:	carbs:		CARDIO	MILES
	D	cal:	carbs:			STEP COUNT
	S	cal:	carbs:		FLEXIBILITY	CALORIES BURNT
MON	B	cal:	carbs:		STRENGTH	DURATION
	L	cal:	carbs:		CARDIO	MILES
	D	cal:	carbs:			STEP COUNT
	S	cal:	carbs:		FLEXIBILITY	CALORIES BURNT
TUES	B	cal:	carbs:		STRENGTH	DURATION
	L	cal:	carbs:		CARDIO	MILES
	D	cal:	carbs:			STEP COUNT
	S	cal:	carbs:		FLEXIBILITY	CALORIES BURNT
WED	B	cal:	carbs:		STRENGTH	DURATION
	L	cal:	carbs:		CARDIO	MILES
	D	cal:	carbs:			STEP COUNT
	S	cal:	carbs:		FLEXIBILITY	CALORIES BURNT
THUR	B	cal:	carbs:		STRENGTH	DURATION
	L	cal:	carbs:		CARDIO	MILES
	D	cal:	carbs:			STEP COUNT
	S	cal:	carbs:		FLEXIBILITY	CALORIES BURNT
FRI	B	cal:	carbs:		STRENGTH	DURATION
	L	cal:	carbs:		CARDIO	MILES
	D	cal:	carbs:			STEP COUNT
	S	cal:	carbs:		FLEXIBILITY	CALORIES BURNT
SAT	B	cal:	carbs:		STRENGTH	DURATION
	L	cal:	carbs:		CARDIO	MILES
	D	cal:	carbs:			STEP COUNT
	S	cal:	carbs:		FLEXIBILITY	CALORIES BURNT

Health Tracker

	WEEKLY MEAL PLAN			WATER INTAKE	WORKOUT/EXERCISE	
SUN	B	cal:	carbs:		STRENGTH	DURATION
	L	cal:	carbs:		CARDIO	MILES
	D	cal:	carbs:			STEP COUNT
	S	cal:	carbs:		FLEXIBILITY	CALORIES BURNT
MON	B	cal:	carbs:		STRENGTH	DURATION
	L	cal:	carbs:		CARDIO	MILES
	D	cal:	carbs:			STEP COUNT
	S	cal:	carbs:		FLEXIBILITY	CALORIES BURNT
TUES	B	cal:	carbs:		STRENGTH	DURATION
	L	cal:	carbs:		CARDIO	MILES
	D	cal:	carbs:			STEP COUNT
	S	cal:	carbs:		FLEXIBILITY	CALORIES BURNT
WED	B	cal:	carbs:		STRENGTH	DURATION
	L	cal:	carbs:		CARDIO	MILES
	D	cal:	carbs:			STEP COUNT
	S	cal:	carbs:		FLEXIBILITY	CALORIES BURNT
THUR	B	cal:	carbs:		STRENGTH	DURATION
	L	cal:	carbs:		CARDIO	MILES
	D	cal:	carbs:			STEP COUNT
	S	cal:	carbs:		FLEXIBILITY	CALORIES BURNT
FRI	B	cal:	carbs:		STRENGTH	DURATION
	L	cal:	carbs:		CARDIO	MILES
	D	cal:	carbs:			STEP COUNT
	S	cal:	carbs:		FLEXIBILITY	CALORIES BURNT
SAT	B	cal:	carbs:		STRENGTH	DURATION
	L	cal:	carbs:		CARDIO	MILES
	D	cal:	carbs:			STEP COUNT
	S	cal:	carbs:		FLEXIBILITY	CALORIES BURNT

Health Tracker

	WEEKLY MEAL PLAN			WATER INTAKE	WORKOUT/EXERCISE	
SUN	B	cal:	carbs:		STRENGTH	DURATION
	L	cal:	carbs:		CARDIO	MILES
	D	cal:	carbs:			STEP COUNT
	S	cal:	carbs:		FLEXIBILITY	CALORIES BURNT
MON	B	cal:	carbs:		STRENGTH	DURATION
	L	cal:	carbs:		CARDIO	MILES
	D	cal:	carbs:			STEP COUNT
	S	cal:	carbs:		FLEXIBILITY	CALORIES BURNT
TUES	B	cal:	carbs:		STRENGTH	DURATION
	L	cal:	carbs:		CARDIO	MILES
	D	cal:	carbs:			STEP COUNT
	S	cal:	carbs:		FLEXIBILITY	CALORIES BURNT
WED	B	cal:	carbs:		STRENGTH	DURATION
	L	cal:	carbs:		CARDIO	MILES
	D	cal:	carbs:			STEP COUNT
	S	cal:	carbs:		FLEXIBILITY	CALORIES BURNT
THUR	B	cal:	carbs:		STRENGTH	DURATION
	L	cal:	carbs:		CARDIO	MILES
	D	cal:	carbs:			STEP COUNT
	S	cal:	carbs:		FLEXIBILITY	CALORIES BURNT
FRI	B	cal:	carbs:		STRENGTH	DURATION
	L	cal:	carbs:		CARDIO	MILES
	D	cal:	carbs:			STEP COUNT
	S	cal:	carbs:		FLEXIBILITY	CALORIES BURNT
SAT	B	cal:	carbs:		STRENGTH	DURATION
	L	cal:	carbs:		CARDIO	MILES
	D	cal:	carbs:			STEP COUNT
	S	cal:	carbs:		FLEXIBILITY	CALORIES BURNT

Health Tracker

	WEEKLY MEAL PLAN			WATER INTAKE	WORKOUT/EXERCISE	
SUN	B	cal:	carbs:		STRENGTH	DURATION
	L	cal:	carbs:		CARDIO	MILES
	D	cal:	carbs:			STEP COUNT
	S	cal:	carbs:		FLEXIBILITY	CALORIES BURNT
MON	B	cal:	carbs:		STRENGTH	DURATION
	L	cal:	carbs:		CARDIO	MILES
	D	cal:	carbs:			STEP COUNT
	S	cal:	carbs:		FLEXIBILITY	CALORIES BURNT
TUES	B	cal:	carbs:		STRENGTH	DURATION
	L	cal:	carbs:		CARDIO	MILES
	D	cal:	carbs:			STEP COUNT
	S	cal:	carbs:		FLEXIBILITY	CALORIES BURNT
WED	B	cal:	carbs:		STRENGTH	DURATION
	L	cal:	carbs:		CARDIO	MILES
	D	cal:	carbs:			STEP COUNT
	S	cal:	carbs:		FLEXIBILITY	CALORIES BURNT
THUR	B	cal:	carbs:		STRENGTH	DURATION
	L	cal:	carbs:		CARDIO	MILES
	D	cal:	carbs:			STEP COUNT
	S	cal:	carbs:		FLEXIBILITY	CALORIES BURNT
FRI	B	cal:	carbs:		STRENGTH	DURATION
	L	cal:	carbs:		CARDIO	MILES
	D	cal:	carbs:			STEP COUNT
	S	cal:	carbs:		FLEXIBILITY	CALORIES BURNT
SAT	B	cal:	carbs:		STRENGTH	DURATION
	L	cal:	carbs:		CARDIO	MILES
	D	cal:	carbs:			STEP COUNT
	S	cal:	carbs:		FLEXIBILITY	CALORIES BURNT

Health Tracker

	WEEKLY MEAL PLAN			WATER INTAKE	WORKOUT/EXERCISE	
SUN	B	cal:	carbs:		STRENGTH	DURATION
	L	cal:	carbs:		CARDIO	MILES
	D	cal:	carbs:			STEP COUNT
	S	cal:	carbs:		FLEXIBILITY	CALORIES BURNT
MON	B	cal:	carbs:		STRENGTH	DURATION
	L	cal:	carbs:		CARDIO	MILES
	D	cal:	carbs:			STEP COUNT
	S	cal:	carbs:		FLEXIBILITY	CALORIES BURNT
TUES	B	cal:	carbs:		STRENGTH	DURATION
	L	cal:	carbs:		CARDIO	MILES
	D	cal:	carbs:			STEP COUNT
	S	cal:	carbs:		FLEXIBILITY	CALORIES BURNT
WED	B	cal:	carbs:		STRENGTH	DURATION
	L	cal:	carbs:		CARDIO	MILES
	D	cal:	carbs:			STEP COUNT
	S	cal:	carbs:		FLEXIBILITY	CALORIES BURNT
THUR	B	cal:	carbs:		STRENGTH	DURATION
	L	cal:	carbs:		CARDIO	MILES
	D	cal:	carbs:			STEP COUNT
	S	cal:	carbs:		FLEXIBILITY	CALORIES BURNT
FRI	B	cal:	carbs:		STRENGTH	DURATION
	L	cal:	carbs:		CARDIO	MILES
	D	cal:	carbs:			STEP COUNT
	S	cal:	carbs:		FLEXIBILITY	CALORIES BURNT
SAT	B	cal:	carbs:		STRENGTH	DURATION
	L	cal:	carbs:		CARDIO	MILES
	D	cal:	carbs:			STEP COUNT
	S	cal:	carbs:		FLEXIBILITY	CALORIES BURNT

"YOU DON'T NEED PERMISSION. YOU NEED COMMITMENT".

Health Tracker

	WEEKLY MEAL PLAN	WATER INTAKE	WORKOUT/EXERCISE
SUN	B cal: carbs: L cal: carbs: D cal: carbs: S cal: carbs:		STRENGTH CARDIO FLEXIBILITY DURATION MILES STEP COUNT CALORIES BURNT
MON	B cal: carbs: L cal: carbs: D cal: carbs: S cal: carbs:		STRENGTH CARDIO FLEXIBILITY DURATION MILES STEP COUNT CALORIES BURNT
TUES	B cal: carbs: L cal: carbs: D cal: carbs: S cal: carbs:		STRENGTH CARDIO FLEXIBILITY DURATION MILES STEP COUNT CALORIES BURNT
WED	B cal: carbs: L cal: carbs: D cal: carbs: S cal: carbs:		STRENGTH CARDIO FLEXIBILITY DURATION MILES STEP COUNT CALORIES BURNT
THUR	B cal: carbs: L cal: carbs: D cal: carbs: S cal: carbs:		STRENGTH CARDIO FLEXIBILITY DURATION MILES STEP COUNT CALORIES BURNT
FRI	B cal: carbs: L cal: carbs: D cal: carbs: S cal: carbs:		STRENGTH CARDIO FLEXIBILITY DURATION MILES STEP COUNT CALORIES BURNT
SAT	B cal: carbs: L cal: carbs: D cal: carbs: S cal: carbs:		STRENGTH CARDIO FLEXIBILITY DURATION MILES STEP COUNT CALORIES BURNT

Health Tracker

	WEEKLY MEAL PLAN			WATER INTAKE	WORKOUT/EXERCISE	
SUN	B	cal:	carbs:		STRENGTH	DURATION
	L	cal:	carbs:		CARDIO	MILES
	D	cal:	carbs:			STEP COUNT
	S	cal:	carbs:		FLEXIBILITY	CALORIES BURNT
MON	B	cal:	carbs:		STRENGTH	DURATION
	L	cal:	carbs:		CARDIO	MILES
	D	cal:	carbs:			STEP COUNT
	S	cal:	carbs:		FLEXIBILITY	CALORIES BURNT
TUES	B	cal:	carbs:		STRENGTH	DURATION
	L	cal:	carbs:		CARDIO	MILES
	D	cal:	carbs:			STEP COUNT
	S	cal:	carbs:		FLEXIBILITY	CALORIES BURNT
WED	B	cal:	carbs:		STRENGTH	DURATION
	L	cal:	carbs:		CARDIO	MILES
	D	cal:	carbs:			STEP COUNT
	S	cal:	carbs:		FLEXIBILITY	CALORIES BURNT
THUR	B	cal:	carbs:		STRENGTH	DURATION
	L	cal:	carbs:		CARDIO	MILES
	D	cal:	carbs:			STEP COUNT
	S	cal:	carbs:		FLEXIBILITY	CALORIES BURNT
FRI	B	cal:	carbs:		STRENGTH	DURATION
	L	cal:	carbs:		CARDIO	MILES
	D	cal:	carbs:			STEP COUNT
	S	cal:	carbs:		FLEXIBILITY	CALORIES BURNT
SAT	B	cal:	carbs:		STRENGTH	DURATION
	L	cal:	carbs:		CARDIO	MILES
	D	cal:	carbs:			STEP COUNT
	S	cal:	carbs:		FLEXIBILITY	CALORIES BURNT

Health Tracker

	WEEKLY MEAL PLAN	WATER INTAKE	WORKOUT/EXERCISE	
SUN	B cal: carbs: L cal: carbs: D cal: carbs: S cal: carbs:		☐ STRENGTH ☐ CARDIO ☐ FLEXIBILITY	DURATION MILES STEP COUNT CALORIES BURNT
MON	B cal: carbs: L cal: carbs: D cal: carbs: S cal: carbs:		☐ STRENGTH ☐ CARDIO ☐ FLEXIBILITY	DURATION MILES STEP COUNT CALORIES BURNT
TUES	B cal: carbs: L cal: carbs: D cal: carbs: S cal: carbs:		☐ STRENGTH ☐ CARDIO ☐ FLEXIBILITY	DURATION MILES STEP COUNT CALORIES BURNT
WED	B cal: carbs: L cal: carbs: D cal: carbs: S cal: carbs:		☐ STRENGTH ☐ CARDIO ☐ FLEXIBILITY	DURATION MILES STEP COUNT CALORIES BURNT
THUR	B cal: carbs: L cal: carbs: D cal: carbs: S cal: carbs:		☐ STRENGTH ☐ CARDIO ☐ FLEXIBILITY	DURATION MILES STEP COUNT CALORIES BURNT
FRI	B cal: carbs: L cal: carbs: D cal: carbs: S cal: carbs:		☐ STRENGTH ☐ CARDIO ☐ FLEXIBILITY	DURATION MILES STEP COUNT CALORIES BURNT
SAT	B cal: carbs: L cal: carbs: D cal: carbs: S cal: carbs:		☐ STRENGTH ☐ CARDIO ☐ FLEXIBILITY	DURATION MILES STEP COUNT CALORIES BURNT

WHO AM I BECOMING, AND WHAT HABITS ARE BUILDING THAT VERSION OF ME?

Health Tracker

	WEEKLY MEAL PLAN			WATER INTAKE	WORKOUT/EXERCISE	
SUN	B	cal:	carbs:		☐ STRENGTH	DURATION
	L	cal:	carbs:		☐ CARDIO	MILES
	D	cal:	carbs:			STEP COUNT
	S	cal:	carbs:		☐ FLEXIBILITY	CALORIES BURNT
MON	B	cal:	carbs:		☐ STRENGTH	DURATION
	L	cal:	carbs:		☐ CARDIO	MILES
	D	cal:	carbs:			STEP COUNT
	S	cal:	carbs:		☐ FLEXIBILITY	CALORIES BURNT
TUES	B	cal:	carbs:		☐ STRENGTH	DURATION
	L	cal:	carbs:		☐ CARDIO	MILES
	D	cal:	carbs:			STEP COUNT
	S	cal:	carbs:		☐ FLEXIBILITY	CALORIES BURNT
WED	B	cal:	carbs:		☐ STRENGTH	DURATION
	L	cal:	carbs:		☐ CARDIO	MILES
	D	cal:	carbs:			STEP COUNT
	S	cal:	carbs:		☐ FLEXIBILITY	CALORIES BURNT
THUR	B	cal:	carbs:		☐ STRENGTH	DURATION
	L	cal:	carbs:		☐ CARDIO	MILES
	D	cal:	carbs:			STEP COUNT
	S	cal:	carbs:		☐ FLEXIBILITY	CALORIES BURNT
FRI	B	cal:	carbs:		☐ STRENGTH	DURATION
	L	cal:	carbs:		☐ CARDIO	MILES
	D	cal:	carbs:			STEP COUNT
	S	cal:	carbs:		☐ FLEXIBILITY	CALORIES BURNT
SAT	B	cal:	carbs:		☐ STRENGTH	DURATION
	L	cal:	carbs:		☐ CARDIO	MILES
	D	cal:	carbs:			STEP COUNT
	S	cal:	carbs:		☐ FLEXIBILITY	CALORIES BURNT

Health Tracker

	WEEKLY MEAL PLAN			WATER INTAKE	WORKOUT/EXERCISE	
SUN	B	cal:	carbs:		STRENGTH	DURATION
	L	cal:	carbs:		CARDIO	MILES
	D	cal:	carbs:			STEP COUNT
	S	cal:	carbs:		FLEXIBILITY	CALORIES BURNT
MON	B	cal:	carbs:		STRENGTH	DURATION
	L	cal:	carbs:		CARDIO	MILES
	D	cal:	carbs:			STEP COUNT
	S	cal:	carbs:		FLEXIBILITY	CALORIES BURNT
TUES	B	cal:	carbs:		STRENGTH	DURATION
	L	cal:	carbs:		CARDIO	MILES
	D	cal:	carbs:			STEP COUNT
	S	cal:	carbs:		FLEXIBILITY	CALORIES BURNT
WED	B	cal:	carbs:		STRENGTH	DURATION
	L	cal:	carbs:		CARDIO	MILES
	D	cal:	carbs:			STEP COUNT
	S	cal:	carbs:		FLEXIBILITY	CALORIES BURNT
THUR	B	cal:	carbs:		STRENGTH	DURATION
	L	cal:	carbs:		CARDIO	MILES
	D	cal:	carbs:			STEP COUNT
	S	cal:	carbs:		FLEXIBILITY	CALORIES BURNT
FRI	B	cal:	carbs:		STRENGTH	DURATION
	L	cal:	carbs:		CARDIO	MILES
	D	cal:	carbs:			STEP COUNT
	S	cal:	carbs:		FLEXIBILITY	CALORIES BURNT
SAT	B	cal:	carbs:		STRENGTH	DURATION
	L	cal:	carbs:		CARDIO	MILES
	D	cal:	carbs:			STEP COUNT
	S	cal:	carbs:		FLEXIBILITY	CALORIES BURNT

Health Tracker

	WEEKLY MEAL PLAN			WATER INTAKE	WORKOUT/EXERCISE	
SUN	B	cal:	carbs:		STRENGTH	DURATION
	L	cal:	carbs:		CARDIO	MILES
	D	cal:	carbs:			STEP COUNT
	S	cal:	carbs:		FLEXIBILITY	CALORIES BURNT
MON	B	cal:	carbs:		STRENGTH	DURATION
	L	cal:	carbs:		CARDIO	MILES
	D	cal:	carbs:			STEP COUNT
	S	cal:	carbs:		FLEXIBILITY	CALORIES BURNT
TUES	B	cal:	carbs:		STRENGTH	DURATION
	L	cal:	carbs:		CARDIO	MILES
	D	cal:	carbs:			STEP COUNT
	S	cal:	carbs:		FLEXIBILITY	CALORIES BURNT
WED	B	cal:	carbs:		STRENGTH	DURATION
	L	cal:	carbs:		CARDIO	MILES
	D	cal:	carbs:			STEP COUNT
	S	cal:	carbs:		FLEXIBILITY	CALORIES BURNT
THUR	B	cal:	carbs:		STRENGTH	DURATION
	L	cal:	carbs:		CARDIO	MILES
	D	cal:	carbs:			STEP COUNT
	S	cal:	carbs:		FLEXIBILITY	CALORIES BURNT
FRI	B	cal:	carbs:		STRENGTH	DURATION
	L	cal:	carbs:		CARDIO	MILES
	D	cal:	carbs:			STEP COUNT
	S	cal:	carbs:		FLEXIBILITY	CALORIES BURNT
SAT	B	cal:	carbs:		STRENGTH	DURATION
	L	cal:	carbs:		CARDIO	MILES
	D	cal:	carbs:			STEP COUNT
	S	cal:	carbs:		FLEXIBILITY	CALORIES BURNT

Health Tracker

	WEEKLY MEAL PLAN			WATER INTAKE	WORKOUT/EXERCISE	
SUN	B	cal:	carbs:		STRENGTH	DURATION
	L	cal:	carbs:		CARDIO	MILES
	D	cal:	carbs:			STEP COUNT
	S	cal:	carbs:		FLEXIBILITY	CALORIES BURNT
MON	B	cal:	carbs:		STRENGTH	DURATION
	L	cal:	carbs:		CARDIO	MILES
	D	cal:	carbs:			STEP COUNT
	S	cal:	carbs:		FLEXIBILITY	CALORIES BURNT
TUES	B	cal:	carbs:		STRENGTH	DURATION
	L	cal:	carbs:		CARDIO	MILES
	D	cal:	carbs:			STEP COUNT
	S	cal:	carbs:		FLEXIBILITY	CALORIES BURNT
WED	B	cal:	carbs:		STRENGTH	DURATION
	L	cal:	carbs:		CARDIO	MILES
	D	cal:	carbs:			STEP COUNT
	S	cal:	carbs:		FLEXIBILITY	CALORIES BURNT
THUR	B	cal:	carbs:		STRENGTH	DURATION
	L	cal:	carbs:		CARDIO	MILES
	D	cal:	carbs:			STEP COUNT
	S	cal:	carbs:		FLEXIBILITY	CALORIES BURNT
FRI	B	cal:	carbs:		STRENGTH	DURATION
	L	cal:	carbs:		CARDIO	MILES
	D	cal:	carbs:			STEP COUNT
	S	cal:	carbs:		FLEXIBILITY	CALORIES BURNT
SAT	B	cal:	carbs:		STRENGTH	DURATION
	L	cal:	carbs:		CARDIO	MILES
	D	cal:	carbs:			STEP COUNT
	S	cal:	carbs:		FLEXIBILITY	CALORIES BURNT

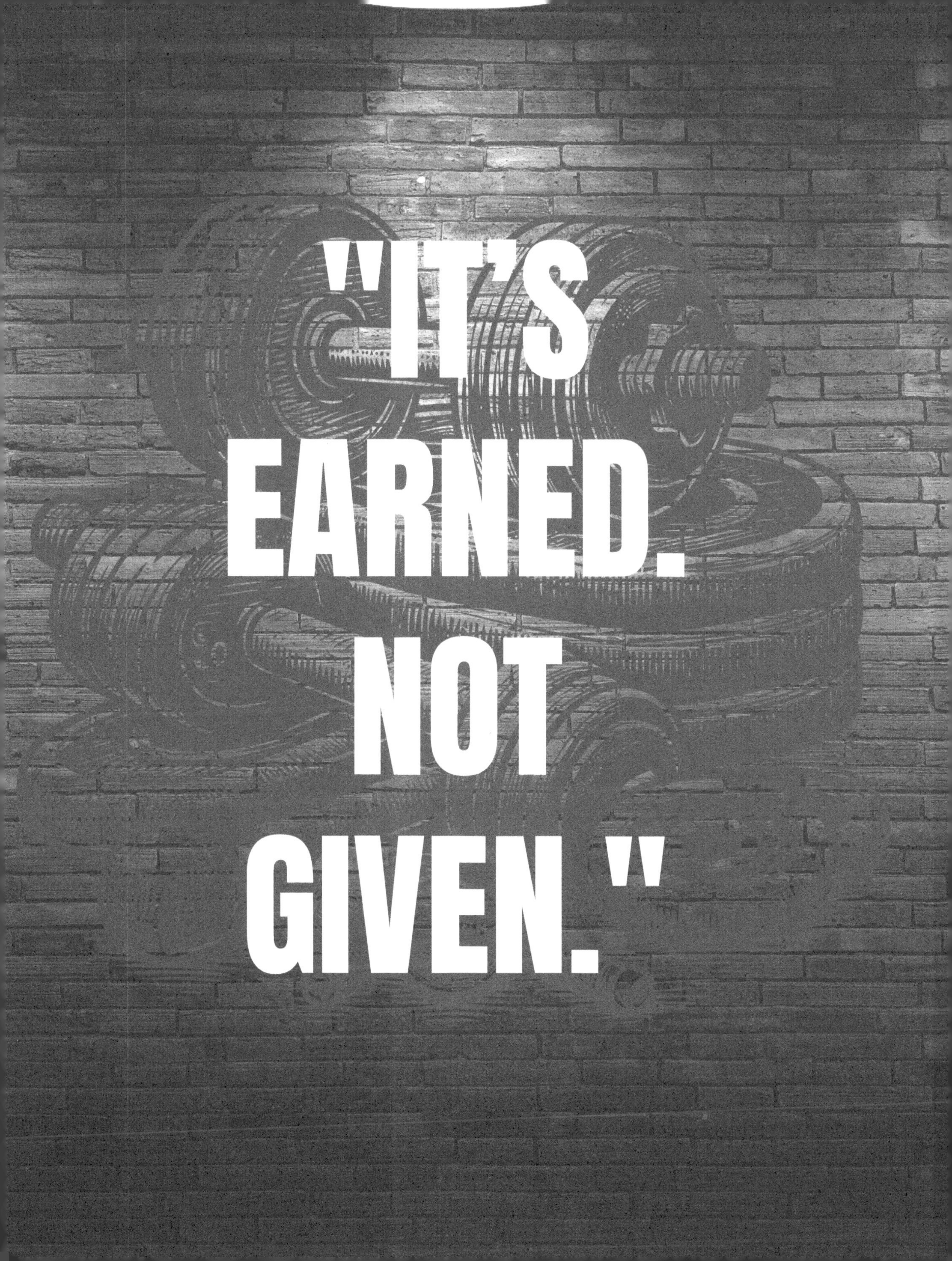
"IT'S
EARNED.
NOT
GIVEN."

Made in the USA
Middletown, DE
05 November 2026

36545524R10077